I0768278

This book is dedicated to my beautiful children, Pharis and Pharaoh.
Seeing you grow brings me a joy I can only describe as love.
Finish whatever you start.
-Love Dad

Table of Contents

Chapter 1
Introduction

Welcome to "The Hardgainer Handbook," a comprehensive guide crafted for those who face the unique challenge of being a hard gainer. If you have ever found it difficult to gain weight, regardless of how much you eat, you are a hard gainer. This term refers to individuals who have a faster metabolism and a naturally leaner physique, making weight gain a challenging feat. But worry not, this book is specifically tailored to turn that challenge into a journey of successful transformation.

Before we get too far into the details, let's get better acquainted with each other. My name is Gabriel Gideon. I'm 6'3" tall, and usually weigh anywhere between 160-170 lbs, and generally feel healthy and well. That's definitely taking a recency-based look at those parameters, because before that I was roughly 148 lbs and had a myriad of health issues.

The struggle to gain weight is often overshadowed by the common pursuit of weight loss. Personally, I found far more resources available for someone looking to lose weight than I did for someone attempting to gain weight. This, for hard gainers, means the journey is equally complex and similarly demands a strategic approach to nutrition and lifestyle. Understanding the crucial role of nutrition in weight maintenance and gain is the first step. Nutrition is not just about eating; it is about eating right. This book will guide you through the nuances of a diet that is high in calories yet rich in nutrients - the kind of diet that fuels healthy weight gain.

In this book, you will be introduced to an array of delicious, high-calorie, high-protein recipes, each designed to cater to your specific dietary needs. Through these recipes, I will help you to understand various aspects of your nutritional needs that will in turn, help you succeed in your weight gain journey. From breakfasts that kickstart your metabolism to dinners that nourish and satisfy, every recipe is an opportunity to enjoy eating while fueling your body. "The Hardgainer Handbook" is more than just a collection of recipes, it's a comprehensive resource that covers everything from the basics of understanding your body's unique needs to practical tips for meal planning and supplement use. You will even find meal plan templates that simplify the process of organizing your diet and insights into how to effectively incorporate supplements like whey and casein for optimal results.

Moreover, we delve into strategies for consistent weight gain, addressing familiar challenges like low appetite and digestive issues, and providing actionable solutions. Each chapter is designed to empower you with knowledge, recipes, and tips to make your weight gain journey not just successful, but also enjoyable. Whether your goal is to bulk up, build muscle, or simply maintain a healthy weight, "The Hardgainer Handbook" is your companion on this path. It acknowledges the challenges you face and offers adaptable, effective strategies to overcome them. So, let's transform the way you eat, live, and thrive.

Chapter 2
Understanding Nutrition

Introduction to Gaining Weight Through Nutrition

Gaining weight is not just about eating more—it is about eating smart. The key lies in understanding and managing your caloric intake versus your caloric burn rate. Calories are the fuel your body needs for energy, and consuming more calories than you burn leads to weight gain. Sounds simple enough.

To truly understand caloric intake though, we must further break this down into macronutrients. The main types we will be concerned with are proteins, carbohydrates, and fats.

Proteins are essential for muscle repair and growth. High-protein foods are a cornerstone of weight gain diets. Some of my personal favorite high protein foods to mix and match throughout my diet are variants of peanut butters, eggs, and sirloin beef. Carbohydrates provide the body with energy. When planning your own meals, choose complex carbs like whole grains that offer sustained energy. I'll usually pair those peanut butters with whole wheat bread. Fats are high in calories and essential for hormonal balance and nutrient absorption. When composing your own meal plans, include healthy fats like avocados, nuts, and olive oil.

This brings me to my final point in the micro-management of our caloric intake. We want to fine tune the smallest details that could give us an advantage in succeeding. For example, olive oil is much better to cook with than vegetable-based oils for our purposes, because it provides us with healthy fats.

Balancing Diet with Exercise

Exercise, particularly strength training, is crucial in ensuring that the weight you gain is muscle, and not just fat. This combination of diet and exercise is essential for a healthy physique. Proper nutrition fuels your workouts and aids in recovery and muscle building.

It's imperative that we understand the differences between different types of workouts, which may do more harm than good. Our focus should be to optimize strength training, with cardiovascular training being minimal. The reason being, that cardiovascular training burns calories at a higher rate. This makes it all to easy to work against our own goals just by running for an extended period.

Tips for Effective Caloric Surplus

- Determine your daily caloric needs based on your activity level and add a surplus to gain weight.
- Have meals and snacks throughout the day to consistently provide your body with calories and nutrients.
- Choose nutrient-dense foods over empty calories to ensure your body gets the right kind of fuel.

Incorporating Supplements for Enhanced Weight Gain

Let's talk about supplements. No, I don't mean the ones you have to take to keep from growing breasts, but supplemental nutrition. These come in the form of shakes usually and can play a pivotal role in your weight gain journey. This becomes especially evident when used in conjunction with a well-planned diet. They are particularly beneficial for hardgainers in filling nutritional gaps and ensuring you meet your daily caloric and protein targets.

Protein Supplements Whey and Casein

Whey Protein is a rapidly absorbed compound, usually in powder form, making it ideal for post-workout shakes for muscle recovery. Casein Protein is a slow-digesting compound, perfect for sustaining muscle protein synthesis when you can't replenish your caloric burn, especially before bed or between meals. Mass Gainers are high-calorie supplements that provide a blend of proteins, carbs, and fats, along with various vitamins and minerals. They are an excellent option for those struggling to consume enough calories through food alone. Add protein powders to recipes (like those in this book) to boost protein content. Use shakes or mass gainers as snacks to maintain a consistent caloric intake throughout the day. Before and after a workout, utilize whey protein to aid in muscle recovery and growth post-exercise.

Understanding and implementing these nutritional principles is the first step towards effective and healthy weight gain. As you explore the recipes in this book, remember that each is designed to align with these principles, helping you on your journey to a healthier, stronger you. With all these various aspects in mind, let us get started.

Chapter 3
Meal Planning

Step 1: Calculate Your Caloric Needs

1. Use the Omni Calculator's Weight Gain Calculator to determine your daily caloric requirement. You can find this calculator online at: https://www.omnicalculator.com/health/weight-gain

 2. Adjust this number based on your personal goals and activity level.

Step 2: Understand Macronutrient Ratios

Step 3: Choose Your Meals

- Breakfast: Select a high-protein option like High-Protein Waffles or Whey-Infused Oatmeal.
- Lunch: Opt for balanced meals such as Protein-Rich Chicken Salad or Protein Bowl.
- Dinner: Choose hearty options like Herb-Grilled Chicken or Vegetarian Chili.
- Snacks and Shakes: Incorporate 2-3 snacks like the Antioxidant Rich Berry Shake or homemade protein bars.

Step 4: Portion Sizes and Meal Frequency

- Divide your total daily caloric intake by the number of meals and snacks to determine portion sizes.
- Consider eating 5-6 smaller meals throughout the day to make calorie consumption easier.

Step 5: Customize and Vary Your Diet

- Use the customization options provided in the book to vary your meals and prevent dietary boredom.
- Ensure you're including a variety of foods to meet all your nutritional needs.

Step 6: Plan and Prep Your Meals

- Allocate time each week for meal planning and preparation.
- Utilize the recipes and tips from the book to prepare your meals in advance.

Step 7: Monitor and Adjust

- Keep track of your dietary intake and adjust your meal plan as needed based on your progress and how you feel.
- Consider keeping a food diary or using a nutrition tracking app.

Chapter 4
Recipes

In "The Hardgainer Handbook," each recipe has been carefully curated not only for its flavor but also for its nutritional value, particularly focusing on the needs of hardgainers. The key to effective weight gain lies in consuming nutrient-dense foods that provide ample calories, proteins, and healthy fats, without compromising on taste and variety. Let's explore the rationale behind the recipe selections and how you can tailor these dishes to your liking.

Breakfast, The Foundation of Your Day

Breakfast sets the tone for the day, providing the initial boost of energy and nutrients. High-protein options like the High-Protein Waffles and Whey-Infused Oatmeal are designed to kickstart your metabolism while providing sustained energy. These meals are rich in complex carbohydrates and proteins - essential for muscle growth and repair.

Customization Options:

• For a vegan twist, use plant-based protein powder and milk alternatives.
• Add nuts or seeds for extra crunch and a boost in healthy fats.

Lunch, A Much Needed Midday Boost

Lunch recipes like the Protein-Rich Chicken Salad and the Protein Bowl are packed with lean proteins and wholesome carbs, ensuring you stay fueled through the day. These dishes are balanced, providing a mix of macro and micronutrients essential for muscle growth and overall health.

Customization Options:

• For the salads, try different protein sources like tuna, tofu, or chickpeas.
• Experiment with various dressings to add new flavors and textures.

Dinner: Satisfying and Nutrient-Rich

Dinner options, including the Herb-Grilled Chicken and Vegetarian Chili, are designed for satiety and nutrient richness. These meals are not only high in protein but also include a variety of vegetables, offering vitamins and minerals crucial for overall well-being.

Customization Options:

• For non-vegetarians, add lean meats like turkey or beef to the Vegetarian Chili.
• Incorporate different herbs and spices to diversify the flavor profiles.

Protein-Packed Snacks and Shakes

Snacks and shakes are integral for maintaining a consistent caloric intake throughout the day. They are easy to prepare and can be a quick source of high-quality proteins and other nutrients. Recipes like the Morning Kickstart Shake and the Antioxidant Rich Berry Shake are perfect for on-the-go nourishment.

Customization Options:

• Mix and match fruits and add-ons like flaxseeds or cocoa powder in shakes for variety and added health benefits.
• Create your own snack bars using the base ingredients of nuts, oats, and your choice of protein powder.

Why These Foods?

The ingredients in these recipes are chosen for their specific nutritional profiles. Foods rich in proteins and healthy fats, like nuts, lean meats, and avocados, are essential for muscle building and providing long-lasting energy. Complex carbohydrates, found in whole grains and starchy vegetables, are vital for sustained energy release. Each recipe balances these nutrients to create meals that are not only fulfilling but also conducive to weight gain and muscle growth.

Adapting to Dietary Restrictions

We understand that dietary needs vary from person to person. That's why each recipe is adaptable. Whether you're vegetarian, vegan, gluten-free, or have other dietary restrictions, you can modify these recipes to suit your requirements. The book provides alternatives and substitutes for various ingredients, making it inclusive for all readers.

The recipes in "The Hardgainer Handbook" are more than just a means to gain weight; they are a pathway to a healthier, stronger, and more energetic life. Each dish is crafted to bring variety, taste, and most importantly, nutritional balance to your meals. Remember, the key to successful weight gain lies in consistency and making informed food choices. Enjoy these recipes, experiment with the suggested variations, and make each meal a step towards achieving your health and fitness goals.

Breakfast Option 1: High-Protein Waffles

Ingredients:

- 1 cup whole wheat flour
- 1 scoop whey protein powder (vanilla or unflavored)
- 1 tbsp baking powder
- 1/4 tsp salt
- 1 egg
- 1 cup milk (or milk alternative)
- 2 tbsp melted unsalted butter or coconut oil
- 1 tsp vanilla extract

Instructions:

1. Preheat your waffle iron.
2. In a large bowl, mix the flour, whey protein powder, baking powder, and salt.
3. In another bowl, beat the egg, and then mix in the milk, melted butter, and vanilla extract.
4. Combine the wet ingredients with the dry ingredients and stir until just blended.
5. Pour the batter onto the hot waffle iron and cook until golden.
6. Serve with your choice of toppings like fresh fruit, yogurt, or honey.

Lunch Option 1: Protein-Rich Chicken Salad

Ingredients:

- 2 cups cooked and shredded chicken breast
- 2 tbsp mayonnaise
- 1/4 cup diced celery
- 1/4 cup raisins
- Salt and pepper to taste

Instructions:

1. In a large bowl, combine the shredded chicken and mayonnaise.
2. Add the celery and raisins. Mix well.
3. Season with salt and pepper to taste.
4. Serve on a bed of greens, in a sandwich, or with whole-grain crackers.

Dinner Option 1: Herb-Grilled Chicken

Ingredients:

- 4 chicken breasts
- 2 tbsp olive oil
- 1 tbsp mixed dried herbs (such as basil, thyme, and oregano)
- 1 tsp garlic powder
- Salt and pepper to taste
- Lemon wedges for serving

Instructions:

1. Preheat the grill to medium-high heat.
2. Rub each chicken breast with olive oil, and then season with mixed herbs, garlic powder, salt, and pepper.
3. Grill the chicken for about 6-7 minutes per side or until fully cooked.
4. Serve hot with a side of steamed vegetables and lemon wedges.

Breakfast Option 2: Protein-Packed Smoothie Bowl

Ingredients:

- 1 scoop whey protein powder (flavor of choice)
- 1 frozen banana
- 1/2 cup frozen berries (blueberries, strawberries, etc.)
- 1/2 cup yogurt
- 1/4 cup milk (or milk alternative)
- Toppings: sliced fruit, nuts, granola, chia seeds

Instructions:

1. In a blender, combine the protein powder, frozen banana, frozen berries, Greek yogurt, and milk.
2. Blend until smooth and creamy.
3. Pour the smoothie into a bowl and add your preferred toppings.
4. Enjoy immediately for a refreshing and protein-rich breakfast.

Lunch Option 2: Protein Bowl with Beans, Sweet Potato, & Whey Protein

Ingredients:
- 1 cup cooked quinoa or brown rice
- 1/2 cup black beans, cooked and drained
- 1 medium sweet potato, diced and roasted
- 1 scoop whey protein powder (unflavored or mildly flavored)
- 1/2 avocado, sliced
- 1/4 cup corn
- Salt, pepper, and spices to taste
- Optional: lime wedges for serving

Instructions:
1. Preheat the oven to 400°F (200°C). Toss the diced sweet potato in a bit of olive oil, salt, and pepper. Roast for 20-25 minutes until tender.
2. Prepare the quinoa or brown rice as per package instructions.
3. Once the sweet potato is done, mix in the whey protein powder while it is still warm.
4. Assemble the bowl: start with a base of quinoa or rice, add the black beans, protein-infused sweet potato, avocado, and corn.
5. Season with salt, pepper, and spices.
6. Serve with lime wedges for an extra zing.

Dinner Option 2: Protein-Packed Turkey Burgers

Ingredients:

- 1 pound ground turkey
- 1 scoop whey protein powder (unflavored)
- 1 egg
- 1/4 cup breadcrumbs
- 1/2 onion, finely chopped
- 1 clove garlic, minced
- Salt and pepper to taste
- Whole-grain buns and toppings (lettuce, tomato, cheese)

Instructions:

1. In a large bowl, mix the ground turkey, whey protein powder, egg, breadcrumbs, onion, garlic, salt, and pepper.
2. Form the mixture into patties.
3. Grill or pan-fry the patties over medium heat for about 5 minutes on each side or until cooked through.
4. Serve on whole-grain buns with your choice of toppings.

Breakfast Option 3: Whey-Infused Oatmeal

Ingredients:

* 1 cup rolled oats
* 1 scoop whey protein powder (flavor of choice)
* 2 cups water or milk (for a creamier texture)
* Pinch of salt
* Toppings: Fresh fruits, nuts, honey, or maple syrup

Instructions:

1. In a saucepan, bring the water or milk to a boil. Add a pinch of salt.
2. Stir in the oats and reduce heat to a simmer. Cook for about 5 minutes, stirring occasionally.
3. Once the oats are cooked, remove from heat, and stir in the whey protein powder until well combined.
4. Serve in a bowl and add your choice of toppings.

Lunch Option 3: Beef and Broccoli Stir-Fry with Whey

Ingredients:

- 1 pound beef, thinly sliced (suitable for stir-fry)
- 1 scoop whey protein powder (unflavored or beef flavored)
- 2 cups broccoli florets
- 1 onion, sliced
- 2 cloves garlic, minced
- 2 tbsp soy sauce
- 1 tbsp sesame oil
- 1 tsp cornstarch
- Salt and pepper to taste
- Optional: Serve with brown rice or quinoa

Instructions:

1.   In a bowl, mix the cornstarch and whey protein powder with soy sauce to create a marinade. Add the beef slices, coat them well, and set aside for 15 minutes.
2.   Heat the sesame oil in a wok or large skillet over medium-high heat. Add the garlic and onion, sautéing until fragrant.
3.   Add the marinated beef and stir-fry until it is nearly cooked through.
4.   Add the broccoli florets, continuing to stir-fry until the beef is fully cooked and the broccoli is tender yet crisp.
5.   Season with salt and pepper, and serve hot, optionally over brown rice or quinoa.

Dinner Option 3: Grilled Salmon

Ingredients:

- 4 salmon fillets
- 2 tbsp olive oil
- 1 lemon) for fresh juice)
- 2 cloves garlic, minced
- Salt and pepper to taste
- Optional: Fresh herbs for garnish (dill or parsley)

Instructions:

1. Preheat the grill to medium-high heat.
2. In a small bowl, mix the olive oil, lemon juice, and minced garlic.
3. Brush the salmon fillets with the lemon and garlic mixture, then season with salt and pepper.
4. Grill the salmon for about 4-5 minutes on each side or until cooked to your liking.
5. Garnish with fresh herbs and serve with a side of steamed vegetables or a salad.

Breakfast Option 4: Scrambled Eggs with Whey Protein

Ingredients:
- 4 large eggs
- 1 scoop whey protein powder (unflavored or mildly flavored)
- 2 tbsp milk or milk alternative
- Salt and pepper to taste
- 1 tbsp butter or olive oil
- Optional: chopped vegetables (spinach, tomatoes, bell peppers), shredded cheese

Instructions:
1. In a bowl, whisk together the eggs, whey protein powder, milk, salt, and pepper until well combined.
2. Heat butter or oil in a non-stick skillet over medium heat.
3. Pour in the egg mixture and let it sit, without stirring, for 20 seconds. Add vegetables or cheese if desired.
4. Gently scramble the eggs, folding them over from the edges to the center until they are softly set and slightly runny in places.
5. Remove from the heat and let them finish cooking in the residual heat of the pan.

Lunch Option 4: Grilled Cheese with Whey Protein Bread

Ingredients for Whey Protein Bread:
- 1 cup oat flour
- 2 scoops whey protein powder (unflavored or vanilla)
- 1 tsp baking powder
- 1/2 tsp salt
- 4 egg whites
- 1/2 cup Greek yogurt

For the Grilled Cheese:
- Whey protein bread slices
- Cheese slices of your choice
- Butter or olive oil for grilling

Instructions:
1. For the Bread: Preheat the oven to 350°F (175°C). Mix oat flour, whey protein powder, baking powder, and salt in a bowl. In another bowl, whisk egg whites and Greek yogurt, then combine with the dry ingredients. Pour into a loaf pan and bake for 20-25 minutes. Let it cool and slice.
2. For the Grilled Cheese: Heat a skillet over medium heat. Butter one side of each bread slice. Place one slice, buttered side down, in the skillet. Add cheese and top with another slice, buttered side up. Cook until golden brown on both sides.

Dinner Option 4: Vegetarian Chili with Whey Protein

Ingredients:

- 1 scoop whey protein powder (unflavored)
- 1 can black beans, drained and rinsed
- 1 can of kidney beans, drained and rinsed
- 1 can diced tomatoes
- 1 onion, chopped
- 2 cloves garlic, minced
- 1 bell pepper, chopped
- 2 tsp chili powder
- 1 tsp cumin
- Salt and pepper to taste
- Optional: sour cream, shredded cheese, fresh cilantro for garnish

Instructions:

1.   In a large pot, sauté onion, garlic, and bell pepper until softened.
2.   Add black beans, kidney beans, and diced tomatoes (with their juice). Stir in chili powder, cumin, salt, and pepper.
3.   Simmer for about 30 minutes, stirring occasionally.
4.   Before serving, stir in the whey protein powder until well combined.
5.   Serve hot, garnished with sour cream, shredded cheese, and cilantro if desired.

Breakfast Option 5: Protein Yogurt Parfait

Ingredients:

- 1 cup yogurt
- 1 scoop whey protein powder (vanilla or a flavor of your choice)
- 1/2 cup granola
- 1/2 cup mixed berries (strawberries, blueberries, raspberries)
- Optional: honey or maple syrup for sweetness

Instructions:

1. In a bowl, mix the yogurt with the whey protein powder until well combined.
2. In a serving glass or bowl, layer the yogurt mixture, granola, and mixed berries.
3. Repeat the layers until all ingredients are used.
4. Drizzle with honey or maple syrup if desired.

Lunch Option 5: Tuna Salad with Whey Protein Bread

Ingredients:
- 1 can of tuna, drained
- 1/4 cup Greek yogurt or mayonnaise
- 1/4 cup diced celery
- 1/4 cup diced apple
- Salt and pepper to taste
- Lemon juice to taste

Ingredients for Whey Protein Bread:
- [Refer to the Whey Protein Bread recipe from the previous section]

Instructions:
1. In a bowl, mix the tuna and mayonnaise. Season with salt, pepper, and a squeeze of lemon juice.
2. Serve the tuna salad with a slice on whey protein bread from our previous recipe.

Dinner Option 5: Grilled Steak

Ingredients:

- 2 ribeye or sirloin steaks (about 1-inch thick)
- 2 tbsp olive oil
- Salt and pepper to taste
- Optional: garlic powder, dried herbs (thyme, rosemary)

Instructions:

1. Allow steaks to come to room temperature (about 20 minutes before cooking).
2. Preheat the grill or skillet to high heat.
3. Rub each steak with olive oil and season generously with salt, pepper, and optional spices.
4. Grill or pan-sear the steaks for 4-5 minutes on each side for medium-rare, or longer for desired doneness.
5. Let the steaks rest for a few minutes before serving.

Chapter 5
Supplements & Shakes

There are practical aspects of incorporating supplements like whey protein, casein, and mass gainers into daily diets. Tailoring supplement use is based on individual dietary requirements and fitness goals. Determine the best times to consume diverse types of supplements (e.g., whey protein post-workout, casein before bed). Incorporate protein powders into regular meals, such as mixing whey into oatmeal or yogurt, or using protein powders in baking.

Quick Recipes for Homemade Nutrition Shakes

Morning Kickstart Shake
*   Ingredients: Whey protein, cold coffee, banana, almond milk, a teaspoon of cinnamon.
*   Instructions: Blend all ingredients until smooth.
*   Optimal Timing: Ideal for breakfast or an early morning snack, providing energy boosts.

Post-Workout Recovery Shake
*   Ingredients: Whey protein, coconut water, frozen berries, and a handful of spinach.
*   Instructions: Blend until smooth.
*   Optimal Timing: Best consumed immediately after a workout for muscle recovery and replenishment.

Soothing Casein Night Shake
*   Ingredients: Casein protein, almond milk, almond butter, pinch of nutmeg.
*   Instructions: Blend until creamy.
*   Optimal Timing: Perfect as a pre-bedtime snack to support overnight muscle repair and growth.

Midday Energy Booster Shake
*   Ingredients: Whey protein, a shot of espresso, banana, Greek yogurt, honey.
*   Instructions: Combine all ingredients and blend until smooth.
*   Optimal Timing: Great for a midday pick-me-up, especially on workout days.
Antioxidant-Rich Berry Shake
*   Ingredients: Whey or plant-based protein, mixed berries, spinach, flaxseed, milk, or juice.
*   Instructions: Blend all ingredients thoroughly.
*   Optimal Timing: Suitable for any time of the day, packed with antioxidants and protein.

Tropical Mass Gainer Shake
-     Ingredients: Mass gainer supplement, pineapple chunks, mango, coconut milk, and a scoop of yogurt.
-     Instructions: Blend until you achieve smooth consistency.
-     Optimal Timing: Excellent for a calorie-dense mid-morning or afternoon snack.

Chapter 6
Practical Tips & Tricks

6.1 Strategy for Consistent Weight Gain

Stay in a caloric surplus. Gaining weight fundamentally requires consuming more calories than your body burns in a day. This section will explain how to calculate your daily caloric needs and the importance of maintaining a caloric surplus for weight gain. We will guide how to increase your caloric intake safely and effectively, focusing on nutrient-dense foods rather than empty calories.

Set a daily calorie goal that exceeds your maintenance level by about 500 calories. For instance, if your maintenance is 2,500 calories, aim for 3,000. Include nutrient-dense foods like lean meats, whole grains, and healthy fats in your meals to meet this goal. Use tools like calorie-tracking apps or your phone's notepad to track your intake.

Eat balanced meals. A balanced diet is key to healthy weight gain. The importance of including a mix of proteins, carbohydrates, and fats in every meal is essential. Proteins are crucial for muscle building and repair, carbohydrates provide the energy needed for daily activities, and fats are essential for hormone production and nutrient absorption. You should construct well-rounded meals that support weight gain goals and your activity levels throughout the day.

Create a meal plan that divides your macronutrients effectively throughout the day. For example, breakfast could include eggs (protein), whole-grain toast (carbs), and avocado (fat). Lunch might be grilled chicken (protein), quinoa (carbs), and olive oil dressing (fat). Dinner could be salmon (protein), sweet potatoes (carbs), and a side of mixed nuts (fat).

Commit to frequent eating. For many hard gainers, eating large meals can be challenging. Therefore, we will stress the benefits of eating more frequently throughout the day. This approach not only makes it easier to consume more calories but also helps maintain a constant energy level and supports better nutrient absorption.

Instead of three large meals, aim for 5-6 smaller, balanced meals. For instance, have a mid-morning snack like yogurt with berries after breakfast, and a mid-afternoon snack like a turkey and cheese sandwich post-lunch. This not only makes it easier to consume more calories but also helps in better digestion and nutrient absorption. Between meals would also be an enjoyable time to get in a nutrition Shake.

Commit to *healthy* snacking. Snacking plays a significant role in adding extra calories to your diet. This section will provide ideas for healthy, high-calorie snacks that are both nutritious and satisfying. The list I have developed below includes options like nuts and seeds, nut butter with fruit, cheese with whole-grain crackers, toast, and yogurt with granola, ensuring there are choices suitable for various tastes and dietary preferences.

• Nuts and seeds: Almonds, walnuts, pumpkin seeds, sunflower seeds.
• Nut butter with fruits: Apple slices with peanut or almond butter.
• Cheese and whole-grain crackers.
• Avocado toast on whole-grain bread.
• Yogurt with granola and a drizzle of honey, or plain yogurt with pineapple or peaches.
• Dark chocolate with almonds.
• Dried fruits like dates or apricots.
• Protein or granola bars.

Develop a consistent eating schedule. Creating a regular eating schedule is crucial for consistent calorie intake, especially for hard gainers. This section will offer tips on how to establish and maintain a routine:

Set specific times for meals and snacks and stick to these times every day. Plan a week's menu in advance to avoid last-minute decisions and ensure balanced nutrition. Set reminders or alarms as prompts to eat, especially useful for those who tend to skip meals due to a busy schedule.

Meal preparation can be a notable change for maintaining a healthy diet. Cook in large batches and store portions for future meals to save time and effort. Use versatile ingredients that can be mixed and matched to create different meals throughout the week and store prepped food, labeling them with dates and contents for easy access.

Keeping track of what you eat, and your progress, is vital for understanding what works best for your body. There are innumerable benefits of maintaining a food diary to record daily intake and observe patterns. Introduce various apps that can help track calories, macros, and physical changes. Do regular, weekly, check-ins with oneself to assess progress and make necessary adjustments.

6.2 Dealing with Common Challenges

6.2.1 Appetite Issues

Smaller, More Frequent Meals:

Many people find it easier to eat smaller amounts more frequently rather than consuming large meals. This approach not only makes it easier to meet calorie goals but can also naturally increase one's appetite over time.

- Example Strategy: Instead of three large meals, aim for 5-6 smaller meals. Start with easy-to-eat foods like smoothies or yogurt bowls and gradually introduce more substantial meals.

Appealing Food Presentation:

The way food is presented can have a significant impact on appetite. A well-plated meal can make eating more enjoyable and appealing.

- Visual Appeal: Use colorful ingredients and take a moment to arrange them attractively on the plate.
- Serving Size: Serve food in smaller portions on larger plates. This can make meals seem less overwhelming and more approachable.

Herbs and Spices:

Incorporating a variety of herbs and spices can enhance the flavor of meals, making them more enticing.
- Flavor Experimentation: Experiment with different seasonings to find what excites your palate. For instance, adding cinnamon to oatmeal or paprika to grilled chicken can elevate the taste significantly.
- Gentle on Digestion: Choose herbs and spices that are also known to aid digestion, such as ginger or fennel.

Stay Active:

Regular physical activity is not only essential for health and muscle building but also for stimulating appetite.

- Moderate Exercise: Engage in moderate exercise like brisk walking, cycling, or light weightlifting. This can increase your metabolic rate and hence your appetite.
- Timing: Try to schedule exercise sessions a little before mealtimes to capitalize on the increased hunger post-workout.

6.2.2 Digestive Concerns

Gradual Increase in Intake:

Abruptly increasing calorie intake can be a shock to the system. Gradually increasing food intake allows the digestive system to adapt without discomfort.

•	Example Strategy: Start by adding an extra 200-300 calories to your daily intake and then slowly increase this amount every week. This can be as simple as adding a snack or slightly larger portions to your meals.

High Fiber Foods:

Fiber plays a crucial role in digestion. It helps in maintaining bowel health and preventing constipation, which can be a side effect of a high-calorie diet.

•	Incorporation Tips: Include a variety of fiber-rich foods in your diet, such as leafy greens, fruits like apples and berries, and whole grains like oats and quinoa.
•	Balanced Approach: While fiber is important, too much can also cause digestive distress. Balance is key.

Stay Hydrated:

Proper hydration is essential for digestion, especially when increasing fiber intake.

•	Hydration Tips: Aim for at least 8-10 glasses of water a day. Including hydrating foods like cucumbers, watermelon, and celery can also contribute to your daily water intake.
•	Monitoring Hydration: Pay attention to the color of your urine – it should be light yellow. Darker urine can be a sign of dehydration.
Probiotics:

Probiotics are beneficial bacteria that support gut health and can aid digestion.

•	Food Sources: Include probiotic-rich foods like yogurt, kefir, sauerkraut, and miso in your diet.
•	Supplementation: If dietary sources are insufficient, consider probiotic supplements, but it is advisable to consult with a healthcare provider before starting any supplement.

6.2.3 Plateaus

Reassess Caloric Needs:

As your body changes, so do its nutritional requirements. A weight gain plateau may indicate that your current caloric intake is no longer creating a surplus.

•	Adjustment Tips: Every few weeks, reassess your caloric needs. This can be done using online calculators or consulting with a nutritionist. If you have gained weight, you will need to increase your intake to continue gaining.

Change Up Your Routine:

Our bodies are incredibly adaptable and can become accustomed to a regular workout routine, leading to plateaus.

•	Exercise Variation: Introduce new exercises or change your existing workout regimen. This can mean altering the intensity, duration, or type of exercise.
•	Progressive Overload: Continually challenge your muscles by increasing the weight or resistance in your workouts, encouraging continued growth and adaptation.

Quality Over Quantity:

While increasing caloric intake is essential for weight gain, the quality of those calories is equally important.

•	Nutrient-Dense Foods: Focus on foods that are not only high in calories but also rich in nutrients. Foods like lean meats, nuts, avocados, whole grains, and legumes are great choices.
•	Avoid Empty Calories: Limit foods that are high in calories but low in nutritional value, like sugary snacks and fast food.

Rest and Recovery:

Adequate rest and recovery are crucial components of a successful weight gain plan.

•	Importance of Sleep: Ensure you are getting enough sleep each night, as this is when most muscle repair and growth occur.
•	Active Recovery: Incorporate light activities like walking or gentle stretching on rest days to aid muscle recovery.
•	Listen to Your Body: Pay attention to signs of overtraining, such as persistent fatigue or decreased performance, and adjust your routine accordingly.

Chapter 7
Reference

Nutritional Information in this section is source from the USDA website and is not based on any specific brand or specialty food type. For precise measurement, use the provided values as markers for your own goals given the amount of weight you want to gain and over what period.

1
High-Protein Waffles
Calories: 944 kcal
Protein: 54.44 g
Carbohydrates: 102.08 g (about 3.6 oz)
Fats: 40.24 g

2
Protein-Rich Chicken Salad
Calories: 776 kcal
Protein: 97.7 g
Carbohydrates: 29.7 g
Fats: 31.1 g

3
Herb-Grilled Chicken
Calories: 988 kcal
Protein: 156.4 g (about 5.52 oz)
Carbohydrates: 0 g
Fats: 44.8 g

4
Protein-Packed Smoothie Bowl
Calories: 354 kcal
Protein: 37.8 g
Carbohydrates: 45.6 g
Fats: 4.2 g

5
Protein Bowl (Beans, Sweet Potato, Whey Protein)
Calories: 705 kcal
Protein: 44.4 g
Carbohydrates: 98.0 g
Fats: 17.2 g

6
Protein-Packed Turkey Burgers
Calories: 956 kcal
Protein: 138.4 g (about 4.88 oz)
Carbohydrates: 27.5
Fats: 39.62 g

7
Whey-Infused Oatmeal
Nutritional Information (per entire recipe):
Calories: 720 kcal
Protein: 51 g
Carbohydrates: 81 g
Fats: 22 g

8
Beef and Broccoli Stir-Fry with Whey
Calories: 1018 kcal
Protein: 126.7 g (about 4.47 oz)
Carbohydrates: 32.9 g
Fats: 37.8 g

9
Grilled Salmon
Calories: 1598 kcal
Protein: 177.0 g (about 6.24 oz)
Carbohydrates: 7.4 g
Fats: 104.22 g (about 3.68 oz)

10
Scrambled Eggs with Whey Protein
Calories: 513 kcal
Protein: 49 g
Carbohydrates: 5.5 g
Fats: 33.9 g

11
Grilled Cheese with Whey Protein Bread
Calories: 462 kcal
Protein: 30.62 g
Carbohydrates: 14.3 g
Fats: 31.54 g

12
Vegetarian Chili with Whey Protein
Calories: 1007 kcal
Protein: 78.1 g
Carbohydrates: 173.5 g (about 6.12 oz)
Fats: 3.82 g

13
Protein Yogurt Parfait
Calories: 453 kcal
Protein: 46.5 g
Carbohydrates: 48 g
Fats: 9.2 g

14
Tuna Salad with Whey Protein Bread
Calories: 330 kcal
Protein: 52.82 g

Carbohydrates: 21.1 g
Fats: 3.04 g

15
Grilled Steak
Calories: 1360 kcal
Protein: 156 g (about 5.5 oz)
Carbohydrates: 0 g
Fats: 92 g

9 798882 152399